# SCIATICA EXERCISES & TREATMENT

## (For Beginners & Seniors)

A Step-by-Step Program to Assist Seniors in Managing Back, Sciatica, and Other Pains.

**Title:**

# SCIATICA EXERCISES & TREATMENT

### (For Beginners & Seniors)

A Step-by-Step Program to Assist Seniors in Managing Back, Sciatica, and Other Pains.



Printed in the United States of America.

**ISBN: 9798871174364**

# TABLE OF CONTENT

# Introduction

Sciatica is the term used to describe the symptoms that manifest themselves when the sciatic nerve is compressed into a painful position. Not only is the sciatic nerve the longest nerve in the body, but it also holds the record for having the longest nerve! The lumbar spine is the starting point, and it travels down the leg until it reaches the foot. When it is irritated, it causes pain, numbness, and/or tingling in specific areas of the body. It also has the potential to bring about all three of these experiences.

In many cases, the discomfort that is linked with sciatica can be alleviated by engaging in physical activity. Having said that, it is of the utmost importance to maintain an awareness of the types of physical activities that do not involve any risks. Others can have the opposite effect, making the discomfort even more severe than it already is.

This article will offer you a list of specific activities and exercises that you should avoid if you suffer from sciatica. Additionally, it will give you a list of activities and exercises that are recommended to assist in relieving pain.

# What Is Sciatica?

If a damaged disc in the spine or other tissues exerts a significant amount of pressure on the sciatic nerve, it has the potential to incapacitate the nerve, rendering it unable to perform its typical duties. This syndrome is commonly referred to as sciatica. If something similar takes occurs, the ailment that is brought about as a consequence is known as a compressed or pinched nerve.

It is common for the symptoms of sciatica to start in the lower back and then spread down the leg of the affected individual. The symptoms may also emerge in the foot in different circumstances.

One of the symptoms of sciatica is the following:

- Numbness

- Electric-shock like pain

- Tingling

- Pins and needles

- Burning pain


Listed below are some of the possible factors that can lead to sciatica headaches:

- Spinal stenosis

- Herniated disk

- Tight piriformis muscle

- Misaligned sacroiliac joint.

# What Is The Feeling Of Sciatica Pain?

The pain that is associated with sciatica can manifest itself in several different ways, depending on the underlying cause. The sensation has been described as being similar to being stabbed, fired, or shocked in the body by some individuals. People have used words such as "burning," "electric," and "stabbing" to describe this experience. Still others have used the word "stabbing."

There is a possibility that the discomfort could be temporary, but it is also possible that it will be permanent. The pain that you are experiencing in your leg is often far more severe than the discomfort that you are experiencing in your lower back. Maintaining a seated or standing position for an extended amount of time, rising from a seated position, or twisting your upper body may cause the discomfort to become more severe. A quick and involuntary movement of the body, such as a cough or sneeze, can also make the pain more acute. This is because the movement is not controlled by the individual.

# Exercises To Avoid

In the event that you have discomfort in the sciatic nerve, you should steer clear of the following exercises.

## Bent-Over Row

When performing a weightlifting exercise known as the bent-over row, the muscles in the back, as well as the backs of the arms, are targeted and strengthened. If you do not appropriately perform the task, it may likely cause discomfort in your back and put you in danger of pulling a muscle or getting hurt.

Exercises like the bent-over row have the potential to increase the likelihood that you will develop disc problems, which can make the symptoms of sciatica even more severe. Your spine contains discs that serve as a cushion and a source of support. These discs are located between each vertebra in your spine.

The symptoms of the sciatic nerve may become significantly more severe if you lift a barbell or hand weights in a manner that causes your back to circle.

## Seated Hamstring Stretch

Hamstring stretches are regularly recommended as a treatment for patients suffering from lower back discomfort. However, the sitting hamstring stretch, which is sometimes referred to as the hurdle stretch, results in the sciatic nerve being subjected to strain.

When you are completing this stretch, you should have one leg extended in front of you in a straight line, and the other leg should be bent in such a way that the sole of the leg that is stretched out straight is touching the knee of the leg that is bent. To stretch the hamstring muscle, you should bend over the leg that is standing straight and then bend at the waist. Applying pressure on the sciatic nerves and causing them to stretch, this position irritates the nerves in the sciatic region.

## Forward Bends

It is best to steer clear of exercises that require you to bend forward from the waist, such as touching your toes or the floor while standing. Pain in the back may be a result of this type of workout. One of the most common movements used in Pilates, calisthenics, and yoga is the forward bend. One example of a forward bend would be the downward-facing dog yoga pose, which is also known as the front bend.

## Double Leg Lifts

You can increase core strength by executing exercises on your back that entail simultaneously lifting both of your legs off the ground. These exercises can be performed on your back. Core exercises are effective in strengthening the muscles of the abdominal region and the lower back; but, because they require the lower back to support the weight of the legs, they also have the potential to irritate the sciatic nerve. The disc may become damaged as a consequence of this, which may subsequently lead to discomfort in the sciatic nerve.

**Full Body Squat**

In addition to putting strain on the lower back, squats have the potential to worsen nerve and spinal injuries (as well as other injuries). When you perform squats, you put strain on your thighs and legs, which makes the discomfort that you feel from sciatica in your leg even worse.

## Deadlifts

The straight-leg deadlift and the Romanian deadlift are two examples of exercises that should be avoided by people who suffer from sciatica because they put strain on the hamstrings.

## Straight legged Sit-Ups

Sit-ups performed with the legs extended on the floor place stress on the spine and aggravate tightness in the sciatic nerve. Inflammation and numbness might develop below the waist as a result of this.

## Abdominal Stretches

Doing abdominal stretches, particularly yoga poses like the cobra and cat-cow, puts pressure on the lower back. This has the potential to cause disc degeneration and exacerbate sciatica pain.

## Leg Circles

It is possible that exercises that entail rapidly stretching the hamstring could make sciatica symptoms worse. This is because these exercises cause the hamstring to be stretched beyond its typical range of motion at the time. In addition to being a component of certain Pilates routines, leg circles are also a component of certain yoga poses and workouts that utilize circuit training modalities.

## High Impact Exercises

Certain types of workouts, particularly those that put pressure on the hips and pelvis, have the potential to exacerbate the symptoms of sciatica. It is recommended that you refrain from engaging in activities such as jogging, jumping, high-impact aerobics, and horseback riding.

# Exercises for Sciatica

The following is a list of exercises that may help relieve the discomfort caused by sciatica:

## Low-Impact Aerobic Activity

Not only can low-impact aerobic activity increase circulation, but it also helps release muscles that have become stiff. To get started, it is suggested that you warm up by engaging in low-impact aerobic activity for ten to fifteen minutes. Some examples of such activities include:

- Walking
- Water exercises
- Riding a stationary bike
- Swimming

You may feel a bit stiff or a little sore in your lower back, legs, or hips when you initially start your warm-up. All of this is to be anticipated. Once a few minutes have elapsed, the muscles must start relaxing as well.

The minimum number of times per week that you should participate in an aerobic exercise that has a minimal impact is five, and you should gradually increase the length of time that you spend doing it. Under the condition that you do not experience any discomfort, you should be able to carry out this kind of training daily.

## Strengthening Exercises

Following the completion of your warm-up, you should proceed to perform exercises that focus on your stomach and back muscles. Listed below are some examples of these kind of things:

- Modified plank
- Bridge
- Pelvic tilt

You can go to more difficult core-strengthening activities as soon as you feel comfortable completing these exercises, provided that increasing the difficulty of the exercises does not cause you to experience any discomfort.

Strengthening exercises should be done three or four times a week, but never on consecutive days.

## Stretches

The discomfort associated with sciatica can be reduced by stretching gently; nevertheless, it is essential to adhere to the following rules to guarantee that you are stretching correctly:

♦ Before stretching, you should always get your blood flowing by engaging in some less strenuous aerobic activity.

♦ When stretching, you should avoid doing any exercises that require you to lean forward or rotate your body at the waist.

♦ Try not to exert yourself against your will. If you feel any resistance, you should avoid pushing yourself deeper.

- If you experience any kind of discomfort while completing a certain stretch, you should immediately stop practicing that stretch.

- When the muscles are cold, you should never extend them. You might try applying moist heat for fifteen to twenty minutes before stretching if you are unable to conduct activities that are designed to warm you up.

- What you are doing should be stopped, the muscle should be allowed to relax, and then you should try again if you feel it becoming more tense.

A few examples of stretches that may be beneficial to certain individuals who suffer from sciatica are as follows:

- The knee-to-chest stretch should only be performed once.

- doing a double stretch that goes from the knees to the chest.

- The length of the piriformis muscle increases.

- You should stretch your hamstrings while lying on your back.

# The Benefits of Exercise for Sciatica

It is not uncommon for the symptoms of sciatica to improve on their own over time; however, certain exercises may hasten the healing process during this period. The most essential thing is to gradually raise the amount of activity you are doing, and if you get symptoms again, you should reduce the amount of exercise you are doing. "Symptom-guided" exercise is the term that is used to describe the process that is being discussed in this particular case.

It is feasible to relax the muscles in the lower back and legs by engaging in activities that have little effect and by stretching softly. This will allow the muscles to relax and become more relaxed. Strengthening your core muscles, which are also referred to as your abdominal muscles, is another one of the most important things you can do to treat sciatica. This is because your core muscles are responsible for supporting your spine. When it comes to treating sciatica, this therapy is among the most successful methods.

## Sciatica Risk Factors?

You most likely have a higher chance of acquiring sciatica if you have any of the following symptoms:

♦ Have a current injury or have a history of having a previous injury: In those who have sustained an injury to their lower back or spine, the likelihood of experiencing sciatica is significantly higher.

♦ Have fun with your life: When you age naturally, the bone tissue and disks in your spine will eventually degrade. This is a natural result of the natural process of aging. It is possible that your nerves could be damaged or pinched as a result of the changes and shifts that occur in bone, disks, and ligaments as a natural part of the aging process.

- What is your weight? You can think of your back as being similar to a vertical crane. The muscles that you have are going to serve as the counterweights. When you hold something in front of your body, the weight that needs to be lifted by your spine (crane) is the weight that you are carrying. It is necessary for the muscles in your back, which serve as counterweights, to exert more effort while you are carrying greater weight on your back. This can lead to back strains, back soreness, and other issues that are associated with the back.

- being deficient in a strong core: When you think of your "core," you are referring to the muscles that are located in your back and belly. You will experience an increase in support for your lower back that is proportional to the strength of your core muscles. In contrast to the region surrounding your chest, which is supported by your rib cage, your muscles are the sole thing that can provide support for your lower back.

♦ Have a job that ensures you are constantly on the go and active: There is a possibility that the likelihood of getting low back problems is increased in occupations that need you to move heavy objects or make frequent use of your back. Therefore, employment that forces you to sit for extended periods may also increase the likelihood of this happening.

♦ If you do not adhere to the appropriate body form while lifting weights or engaging in other forms of strength training activities, you may still be at risk for developing sciatica. Even though you are in excellent physical condition and engage in a great deal of physical exercise, this is nonetheless the case.

♦ Diabetes raises the likelihood of nerve damage, which in turn raises the likelihood of experiencing sciatica. If you have diabetes, your chance of nerve injury is raised.

♦ If you are afflicted with osteoarthritis, your spine may sustain damage, and your nerves may be endangered as a result of the condition.

♦ Your risk of having sciatica will increase if you lead a sedentary lifestyle, which includes sitting for extended periods, not engaging in physical activity, and failing to keep your muscles active, flexible, and toned.

◆ Tobacco contains nicotine, which can cause
damage to the tissue in your spine, weaken
your bones, and speed up the degeneration
of your vertebral disks. If you smoke, be
aware of these potential consequences.

# What Causes Sciatica?

In addition to the following, sciatica can be caused by a variety of medical conditions, including the following:

♦ The term "pinched nerve" refers to a situation in which a herniated disk or sliding disk exerts pressure on a nerve root. The majority of persons who have sciatica do so for this reason, making it the most common cause. There is a range of approximately one percent to five percent of people in the United States will suffer from a slipped disk at some point in their lives. They are referred to as disks, and they are the cushioning pads that are located in between each vertebra of the spine. The gelatinous center of a disk can herniate, or protrude, through a weakness in the outer shell of the disk if the disk is subjected to pressure from the vertebrae. If a herniated disk in your lower back causes one of the vertebrae in that region to get compressed, the sciatic nerve may be affected.

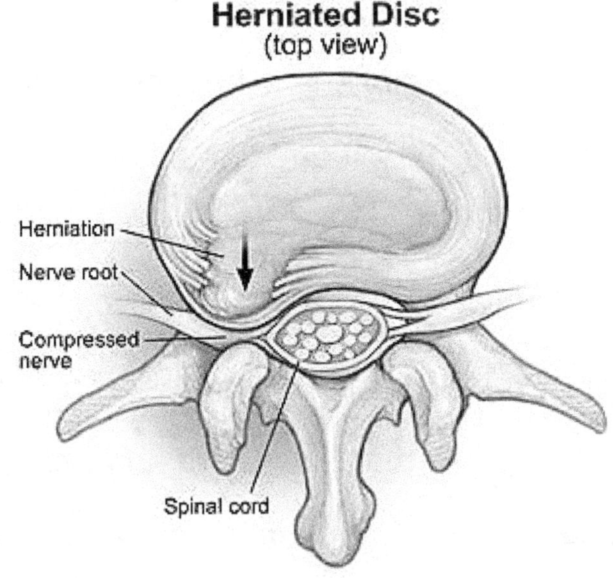



♦ A condition known as degenerative disk disease is characterized by the gradual deterioration of the disks that are situated in the spaces between the vertebrae of the spine. The steady deterioration of the disks leads to a reduction in their height, which in turn causes the neural pathways to become more restricted at the same time (spinal stenosis). Should you suffer from spinal stenosis, the roots of the sciatic nerve may be compressed as they leave the spine.

♦ Spinal stenosis is a condition that occurs when the spinal canal becomes constricted abnormally. It is because of this constriction that there is less space available for the spinal cord and the nerves to move around in that area.

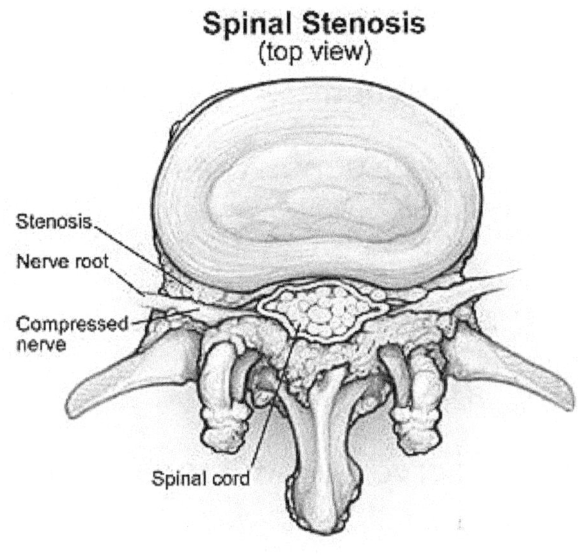



♦ Spondylolisthesis is characterized by the displacement of one vertebra relative to the vertebra above it, which results in a constriction of the canal via which the nerve departs the spinal column. These constrictions the nerve's capacity to travel through the spinal column. The expanded bone in the spine has the potential to cause the sciatic nerve to become compressed.

- Osteoarthritis. As people get older, their spines may acquire bone spurs, which are pointed outgrowths of bone. These spurs can cause nerve compression in the lower back due to their presence.

- A contusion is a type of injury that occurs when the sciatic nerve or the lumbar spine is injured.

- Cancers that form in the lumbar spinal canal and exert pressure on the sciatic nerve are referred to as laminar tumors.

- This muscle, known as the piriformis, is a very small muscle that may be found deep within the buttocks. Piriformis syndrome is a condition that manifests itself when this muscle, which is characterized by spasms or tightness, results in discomfort in the buttocks. This can cause the sciatic nerve to become irritated because it exerts pressure on it. A neuromuscular condition that is not commonly seen is called piriformis syndrome.

♦ A condition known as cauda equina syndrome is a condition that affects the cauda equina, which is a bundle of nerves that is situated at the very end of the spinal cord. This condition is exceedingly rare, yet it has the potential to be fatal. Pain that radiates down the leg, numbness around the anus, and a lack of control over both the intestines and the bladder are all symptoms that are associated with this systemic condition.

## Symptoms Of Sciatica?

The following are some of the symptoms of sciatica:

◆ Pain that ranges from moderate to severe in the buttocks, lower back, and down the affected leg are the symptoms of sciatica.

◆ A feeling of numbness or weakness in your lower back, buttocks, legs, or feet.

◆ Pain that is made worse by movement; immobility as a result of the pain.

◆ Having a sensation similar to "pins and needles" in your legs, toes, or feet.

◆ a loss of control over one's bowel movements and bladder (due to cauda equina).

## Diagnosing Sciatica?

Your medical history will be reviewed first by your healthcare provider. Their next step will be to ask you about your symptoms.

Your doctor or other healthcare provider may ask you to walk during your physical examination so they can see how your spine supports your weight. You may be asked to walk simultaneously on your toes and heels to assess the strength of your calves. Your medical practitioner may also ask you to perform a straight leg lift test. You will be required to lie on your back with your legs extended in front of you for this assessment. One leg at a time, your healthcare provider will carefully elevate each one while noting where you are experiencing pain. This test assists in determining whether or not one of your disks is malfunctioning and helps to pinpoint the affected nerves. To assess the flexibility and strength of your muscles and pinpoint the location of your pain, you will also be required to carry out various stretches and motions.

Depending on what they discover following your physical examination, your doctor may prescribe imaging and further tests. These could consist of the following:

- X-rays of the spine to analyze the patient for any potential fractures, issues with the disks, infections, cancers, and bone spurs.

- Computerized tomography (CT) scans and magnetic resonance imaging (MRI) scans are two imaging techniques that can be used to provide detailed images of the bone and soft tissues of the back. A magnetic resonance imaging (MRI) scan can identify any type of arthritic condition that may be exerting pressure on a nerve, in addition to identifying any type of pressure that is currently present. MRIs are commonly sought by medical professionals to verify a diagnosis of sciatica pain.

- Electromyography and nerve conduction velocity studies are currently being carried out to explore the efficiency with which electrical impulses travel through the sciatic nerve, as well as the response of the muscles inside the structure.

- In order to determine if the pain is being generated by the vertebrae or the disk, a myelogram is performed.

## How Is Sciatica Treated?

This treatment is designed to increase your mobility and reduce the amount of discomfort you are experiencing as a result of your condition. Many cases of sciatica resolve on their own over time with the assistance of some basic self-care techniques. The underlying cause of the condition can vary, but the majority of cases resolve on their own.

The following are some examples of treatments as part of self-care:

The first stage in the process of administering ice and/or heat packs is to apply ice packs to the affected area to alleviate suffering and reduce edema. Ice packs or a bag of frozen vegetables that have been wrapped in a towel should be applied to the affected area to treat it. Twenty minutes of treatment time, numerous times per day, is the suggested duration of treatment. To maintain the temperature of the area beyond the initial few days, you should move to using a hot pack or a heating pad. The time allotted for each application should not exceed twenty minutes. If the pain is still persistent, you can try switching between hot and cold packs to determine which one gives you the greatest relief as you experiment with different combinations.

Medication that is available without a prescription: As a means of accelerating your recuperation, you should use medications that reduce pain, inflammation, and edema. Aspirin, ibuprofen (Advil, Motrin), and naproxen (Naprosyn, Aleve) are just a few examples of the several non-steroidal anti-inflammatory medications (NSAIDs) that are included in this category. Without the need for a prescription, these medications are readily available and can be acquired without a prescription. If you want to take aspirin, you need to exercise extreme caution. The use of aspirin has been associated with some adverse effects, including the development of ulcers and bleeding. As an alternative to nonsteroidal anti-inflammatory medicines, acetaminophen, which is also sold under the brand name Tylenol, is a pain reliever that can be preferred.

After gentle stretching: Through the instruction of an instructor who has experience working with those who suffer from low back pain, you will learn the optimal approach to stretching. You should gradually go to various sorts of strengthening, such as general strengthening, strengthening of the core muscles, and cardiovascular activities.

## When To Seek Medical Attention After Self-Treating Sciatica?

It is possible that the symptoms of sciatica can vary substantially from one individual to the other. There is a wide range of possible manifestations of pain, ranging from minor to severe, and it can arise from several different potential causes. In some cases, it's feasible that the first round of treatment will be more intense. However, in general, if a trial of conservative, self-care treatments such as ice, heat, stretching, and over-the-counter medicines has not provided relief after six weeks, it is time to return to a healthcare professional and try other treatment options. This is because they are more likely to address the underlying cause of the pain. Examples of such therapies include applying ice, applying heat, and stretching.

These are some more therapeutic options that are available:

♦ **Spinal Injections:** A corticosteroid injection, which is an anti-inflammatory medication, could help reduce the discomfort and swelling around the affected nerve roots if it is provided to the lower back in the form of a shot. This would be beneficial for those who are experiencing chronic pain. Pain relief from injections often lasts for up to three months and can be provided as an outpatient treatment while the patient is under the effect of a local anesthetic. Injections can be administered to unconscious patients. You can have a burning or stinging feeling in addition to the pressure that you are experiencing as the injection is being administered to you. Make sure to consult with your healthcare provider about the potential risks that are involved with injections, as well as the maximum amount of shots that you are permitted to have.

♦ **Prescription Medications:** It is possible that your healthcare provider would suggest that you use muscle relaxants to ease the pain that is linked with muscular spasms. Cyclobenzaprine, which is currently available for purchase under the brand names Amrix and Flexeril, is a good illustration of this. Among the several kinds of painkillers that could potentially be studied are tricyclic antidepressants and anti-seizure medications, to name just two examples. You may require prescription medicines at an early stage of the treatment plan; however, this will be contingent upon the intensity of your pain.

♦ **Physical therapy:** The goal of physical therapy is to identify motions of exercise that can alleviate sciatica by releasing pressure that has been exerted on the nerve. This is accomplished through the technique of exercise. Stretching activities, which improve muscle flexibility, should be incorporated into a fitness routine, and cardiovascular workouts should also be included in the routine (such as walking, swimming, and water aerobics). Additionally, your primary care physician may be able to provide you with a referral to a physical therapist. To tailor a stretching and aerobic exercise program to your specific requirements, this therapist will collaborate with you to develop the program. In addition, this therapist will suggest additional exercises that will increase the strength of the muscles in your legs, belly, and back.

- **Alternative therapies:** It is becoming increasingly common to make use of alternative remedies, which are currently being utilized to effectively treat and manage a wide range of pain conditions. Additionally, spinal manipulation performed by a qualified chiropractor is one of the alternative treatment choices for sciatic pain. Yoga and acupuncture are two other alternative treatment methods. It is possible that massage therapy would be beneficial in treating the muscle spasms that are usually associated with sciatica. One of the methods that can be applied to assist in the management of pain and the decrease of stress is known as biofeedback in the medical field.

## The Best Exercises for Sciatica

In the case of sciatica, the National Health Service (NHS) suggests activities that are specifically designed to address the underlying cause (which you will first and foremost need to have determined by your general practitioner). The next step, which you should take once you have that worked out, is as indicated in the following sentence.


If your sciatica is caused by the piriformis muscle, which is a little muscle located in your buttocks, then you should try to stretch out your piriformis muscle by performing the following exercises:

## Exercise 1

➢ When you do this, you should bring your legs in closer to your chest and cross them together.

➢ Hold this position for 10 seconds while pulling your abdominal muscles into a working position.

➢ It is recommended that it be done three times.

## Exercise 2

➢ You should first bring your knees up to your chest, and then you should move them so that they are resting on the shoulder that is opposite the one that is causing you discomfort.

➢ To mobilize and release the piriformis while simultaneously stimulating the abdominal muscles, you should begin by moving your knees from side to side as you are performing this exercise.

**If your sciatica is caused by a herniated or slipped disk, which can cause discomfort locally or along your body, you should try to give the area some space by performing the following exercises for sciatica:**

## Exercise 1

➢ The area will become more open and the pressure will be reduced when you rest on your stomach with two cushions placed under your lower back because of this position.

- Take a few minutes to hold this position before moving on to the next step.

- For the next five seconds, you should make an effort to put as much pressure as you possibly can on your buttocks.

- There should be ten repetitions of this.

**Exercise 2**

- After positioning a pillow in the space between your knees, lie on your side with the side that is causing you discomfort facing upward.

- If you want to relieve strain on your lower back, you should lie on your back and push a pillow or chair between your knees until you are comfortable.

➢ You should gently tilt your pelvis when you are lying on your back.

➢ It is recommended that the lumbar arch in the lower back be pulled down to the floor or bed while holding this position for five seconds.

➢ There should be ten repetitions of this.

**Exercise 3**

➢ For the next five seconds, you should make an effort to put as much pressure as you possibly can on your buttocks.

➢ There should be ten repetitions of this.

*If your sciatica pain is caused by spinal stenosis, you should do the following exercises for sciatica to free up some joint space while simultaneously strengthening and stabilizing the muscles that are around the affected area:*

## Exercise 1

> ➢ When you are lying down on the floor or in bed, bring your knees up to your chest and bring them to your chest.

> ➢ Make ten requests for them to come closer to you.

## Exercise 2

> ➢ Your knees should be brought up to your chest, and then you should move them in circles, first to the side, and then back in both directions. A number of repetitions are required.

➢ Proceed in this manner for a total of ten times around in each direction.

## Exercise 3

➢ If you are sitting on a chair or a bed, you can perform this exercise well. Your knees should be brought up to your chest.

➢ They will benefit from being gently bounced up and down.

## Exercise 4

➢ While you are lying down on the ground or in a bed, you should relax the lumbar arch, which is also referred to as the curvature in your lower back.

➢ There should be ten repetitions of this.

## Exercise 5

> ➤ To perform this exercise, bring your abdominal muscles closer to your spine and roll your knees away from your body.

> ➤ There should be ten repetitions of this.


## Exercise 6

> ➤ Your buttocks should be subjected to some pressure, and your pelvic floor should be pulled toward your spine.

> ➤ For the following five seconds, you should continue to hold.

> ➤ It is recommended that it be done three times.

*In the event that your sciatica is caused by degenerative disc degeneration, you should do the following exercises to strengthen, move, and stabilize the area:*

## Exercise 1

➤ Ensure that your knees are squarely over your ankles by positioning yourself in this manner.

➤ The bridge position is achieved by drawing the buttocks in toward the spine and elevating the pelvis when performing the exercise.

## Exercise 2

➤ Lie on your back on the ground or the bed, bringing your legs up to alleviate pressure off of your lower back, and contract your abdominal muscles.

➢ You should gently tilt your pelvis when you are lying on your back.

➢ It is recommended that the lumbar arch in the lower back be pulled down to the floor or bed while holding this position for five seconds.

➢ There should be ten repetitions of this.

**Exercise 3**

➢ By rotating your knees in a side-to-side motion while lying on your back, you can activate the muscles that are located in your core.

**Exercise 4**

➢ Your pelvic floor should be squeezed whether you are in any position, whether you are standing, sitting, or lying down.

➢ For the following five seconds, you should continue to hold.

➢ You should repeat the process five times.

# In-Bed Sciatica Exercises

Because they can be performed either in the morning or in the evening, exercises for sciatica that can be done in bed can be more useful than other types of exercises.

According to Quinn, you can conduct a variety of exercises while lying in bed. Some of these movements include pulling your knees to your chest, posterior pelvic tilts, and knee to opposite shoulder stretch. The majority of the exercises that are prescribed by the National Health Service (NHS) for sciatica can be completed while lying in bed, and the instructions that are provided above will assist you in identifying when this is an option for you to perform.

# Illustrated Stretches And Exercises For Sciatica

Some of the exercises and stretches that are outlined below may help relieve the discomfort associated with sciatica. You should feel comfortable completing the first three stretches in sequence daily because they are simple and easy to complete. "Let pain be your guide," while you stretch out your muscles. "If things are getting more painful, you might want to change your range of motion so that you are not getting as deep of a stretch," the trainer told the patient. "This will help you avoid getting too stretched."

## ♦ Standing Hamstring Stretch

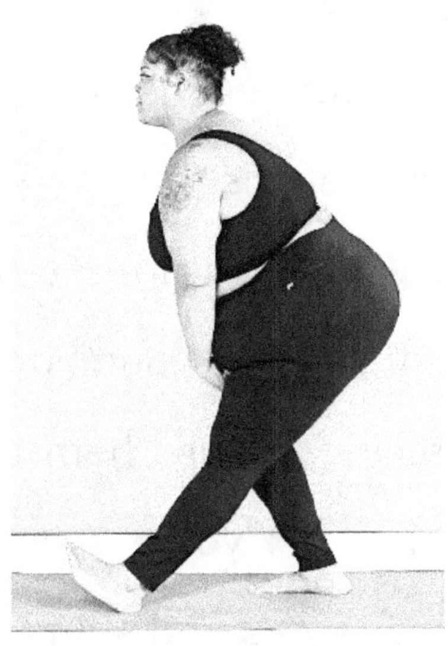

♦ Standing in a comfortable position with your hands at your sides, your core engaged, and your feet hip-width apart is the best way to complete this exercise.

♦ While keeping your left leg straight and flexing it so that only the heel contacts the ground, take a step forward with your left foot.

- Swoop down while keeping your arms straight, bending at the hips, and tracing the length of your leg using your upper body. Raise your hands above your head while standing with your arms straight, and then bring them down to your sides. The sensation of stretching your hamstrings and the lengthening of your spine should occur simultaneously as you stand and stretch.

- Proceed with the opposing foot at this point, and then repeat the process on the opposite side. Switch sides every three to five seconds for the next two minutes; this should be done.

It is expected that this action will result in a significant stretch being applied to the hamstrings as well as the calves, as stated by Scantlebury.

- **Lying Figure Four Stretch**

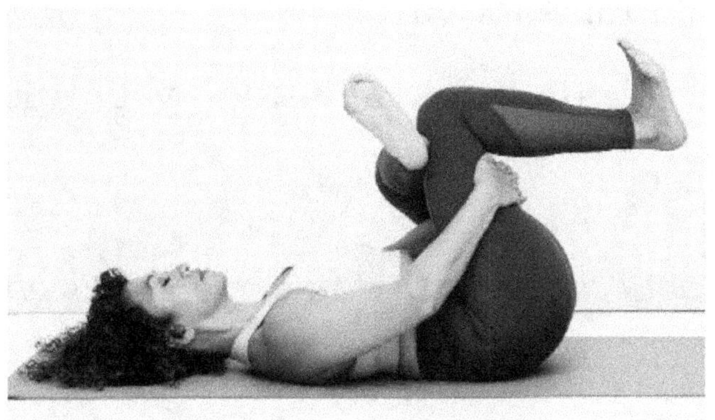

- You should rest your body on your back.

- You need to bend your right knee and move your left foot so that it is crossing over your right quadriceps. In addition, you should move your left foot.

- With your right hand resting on the back of your right leg, draw it in close to your torso and maintain this position.

- You should maintain that position for thirty to forty-five seconds until you have reached a point where you feel a stretch that is comfortable for you.

- After you have adjusted your posture, proceed.

*Scantlebury asserts that this exercise is effective in extending the lateral glute muscles in addition to the piriformis muscles during the activity.*

♦ **Cobra Pose**

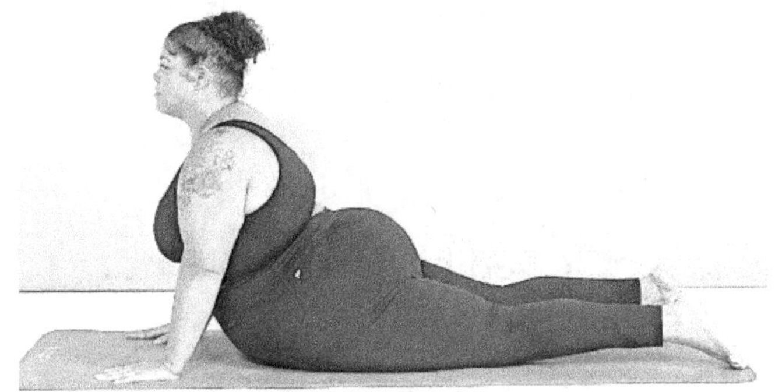

♦ You should lie on your stomach with your palms facing the ground and your hips and chest on the floor. Place your hands slightly below your shoulders and position your palms facing the ground. This is the point at which everything starts.

♦ To lengthen your spine and elevate your shoulders, press through your palms while keeping your hips on the ground. This will help you maintain a stable position. Once you have extended your spine as far as your range of motion will allow, hold the position for one to two seconds at the top of the movement. After that, a brief pause of one to two seconds is followed by a gradual return to the starting posture. It is one repetition.

♦ Continuous repetitions should be performed for a period of two minutes. The range of mobility in your spine should be gradually increased until you reach your goal.

*This particular stretching position, which is frequently used in yoga classes, serves to facilitate the extension of the spine and alleviate pressure on the lower back.*

♦ **Full Cobra pose**

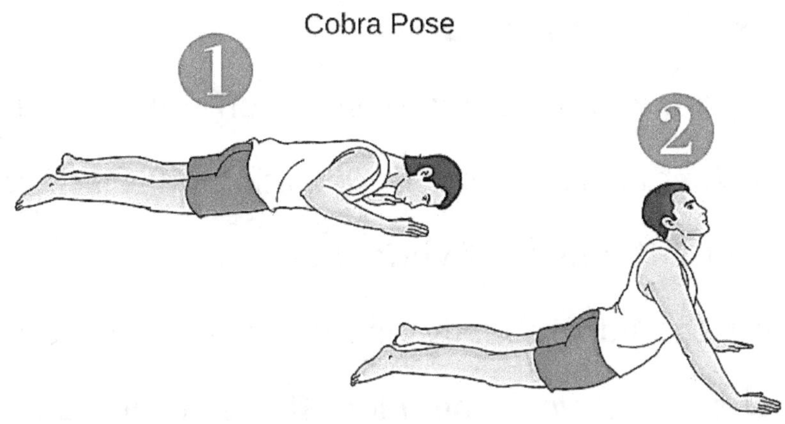

Cobra Pose

- **How it is beneficial:**

When compared to the half-cobra stance, the full-cobra pose provides even greater spinal extension, which helps to press the material of the disc back toward the center of the spine and reduces the pain sensations associated with sciatica. Take caution with this one, and make sure you don't go overboard.

- **How to carry it out:**

- Beginning in a supine position on the ground, place your hands in a flat position on the floor around the level of your shoulders.

- You should gradually apply pressure to your hands to lift your shoulder off the ground until you experience a small stretch.

- By breathing as you press farther into lumbar extension, you can increase the range of motion that you have available to you.

- Aim to complete five repetitions.

- ## Sciatic Nerve Floss

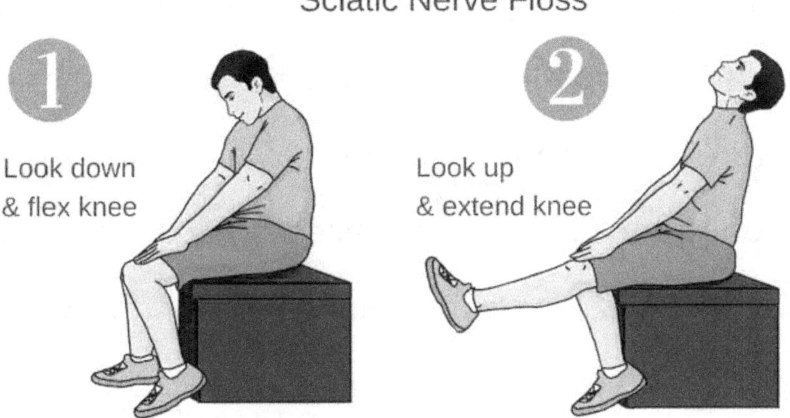


## How it helps:

By massaging the nerve that is trapped, sciatic nerve flossing can be an effective method for relieving lower back pain. When the sciatic nerve is compressed by the muscles, sciatic nerve flossing is performed to "massage" the nerve to relieve the pressure.

**How to do it:**

- One should assume a slouched stance on a chair or table, with both legs falling off the edge of the chair or table.

- Your hands should be placed on your thighs.

- As you gaze up with your head, extend your knee (or straighten it out) and look up.

- At this point, lower your leg while bending your neck down (flexing).

- Return to the spot you started from.

- Twice a day, ten times each.

♦ **Elevated Plank**

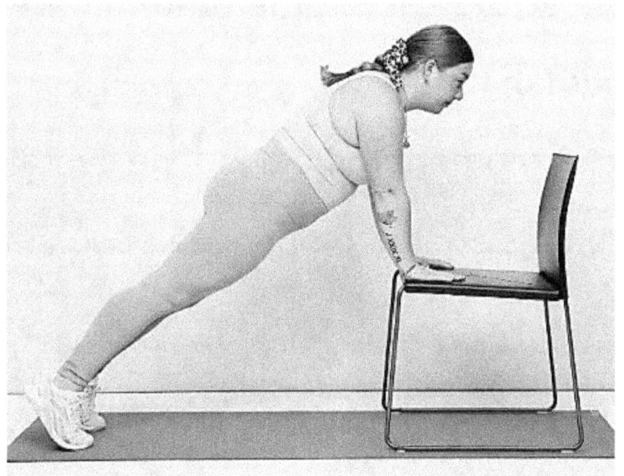

♦ Create a high plank by placing your hands on a sturdy box, stairs, or chair and holding them there. Make sure that your neck is in a neutral position, that your hands are directly beneath your shoulders, and that your vision is fixed ahead of your hands. You should avoid arching your back and make sure that your quadriceps, butt, and core muscles are all tight. Imagine that you are expanding from the top of your head to the bottom of your heels at the same time that you are thinking about length.

♦ Take a moment to hold in. The overall number of rounds should be between two and three.

*When holding the posture, make sure your core feels the majority of the pressure, not your shoulders or back. The higher you raise your hands, the easier the exercise will be. As you become more comfortable with the exercise, try smaller surfaces until you're ready to take on the forearm plank below. If you find that 30 seconds is too long, start with 10- to 15-second holds.*

- **Forearm Plank**

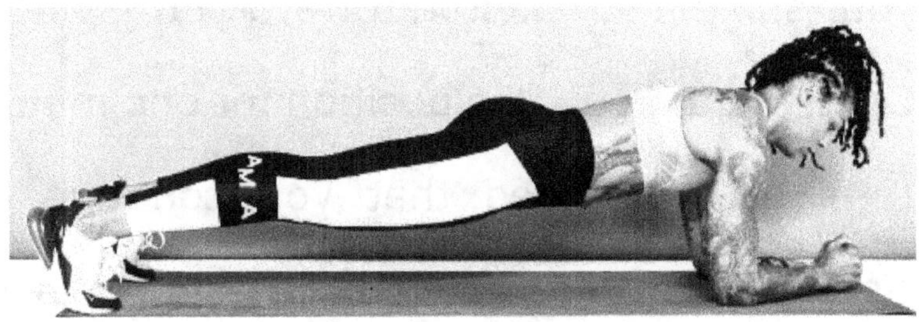

- Your forearms should be placed on the ground, your elbows should be positioned so that they are directly underneath your shoulders, and your hands should be turned so that they are facing forward. Making sure that your arms are in a parallel position is the result of doing this. You should extend your legs behind you and arrange your feet so that they are hip-width apart from one another. With your abdominal muscles, buttocks, and quads engaged, bring your navel in toward your spine and pull it in toward your spine.

♦ Continue to keep this position for one minute. It is recommended that you continue the circuit a total of two to four times after taking rests as prescribed.

*There is a variation of the elevated plank exercise that you may perform at home that is more challenging than this one. Once more, you need to make sure that the majority of the experience is occurring in your abdominal region, rather than in your back or shoulders.*

- **Forearm Side Plank on Knees**

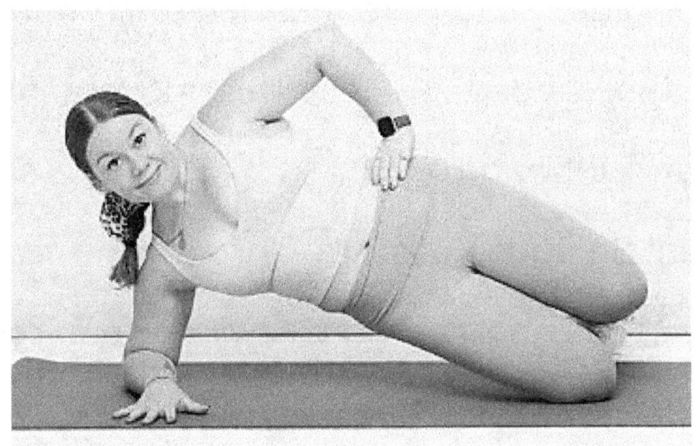

- To complete a kneeling forearm side plank, you should rest your body on your right forearm, stack your elbow below your shoulder, and place your hand in front of your torso. At the same time that you are extending your legs and keeping both knees bent, position your left knee so that it is on top of your right knee.

- Put your left hand on your hip and engage your glutes and core muscles to lift your hips off the ground. Repeat this movement with your right hand.

- Maintain this posture for thirty seconds. Repeat for an additional two to four rounds, pausing after each round as required.

*In addition to teaching you how to appropriately align your spine and contract the front of your core, this strength-training exercise can also teach you how to reduce the amount of back compression you experience. Start with holds that last between 10 and 15 seconds if you find that 30 seconds is too tough.*

## ◆ Forearm Side Plank

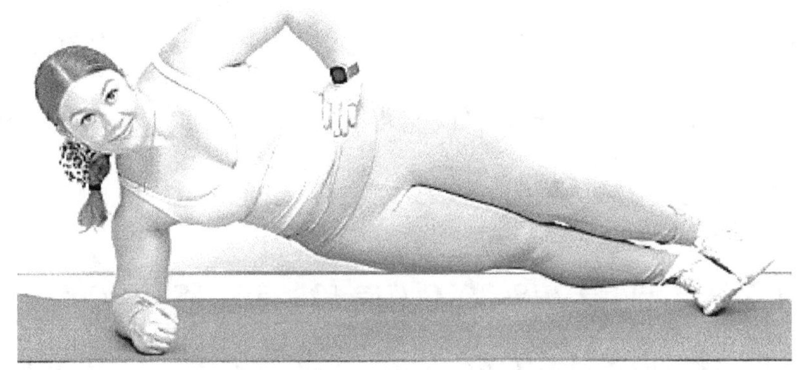

- As you enter a forearm side plank posture, place your right forearm in front of your body to provide support for it. At the same time, stack your elbow beneath your shoulder and place your hand in front of your body. Following the extension of your legs and the placement of your left foot on top of your right, you should then lift your hips off the ground by contracting your abdominal muscles and glutes. It is recommended that you use your left hand to support your hip.

- Maintain this posture for thirty seconds. Repeat for an additional two to four rounds, pausing after each round as required.

*After you have mastered the forearm side plank on the knees, you should make this exercise more challenging for yourself. Immediately following the completion of the planking phase, you should try the door handle squat. Perform ten to fifteen repetitions of this exercise, and then repeat it for three to four rounds.*

- **Bird-Dog Pose**

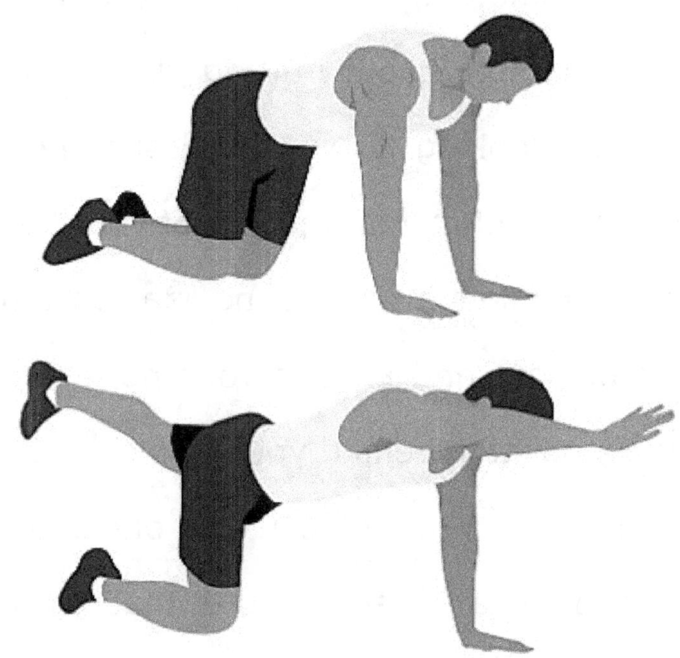

- **How to try it:**

- Make a start on all fours. Make certain that your hands are positioned just below your shoulders and that your knees are positioned directly below your hips.

- As you do so, bring your belly button closer to your spine and engage your core muscles. If you want to avoid putting strain on your neck, try looking forward and slightly down (approximately a foot in front of your hands).

- Raise your left arm in a neutral position in front of you, and extend your right leg in a neutral position behind you. This can be done simultaneously, or you can do it one at a time, and then the other. Ensure that they are properly aligned with your back in a straight line. It may be simpler to examine your form if you do this activity while standing close to a mirror.

- After pausing, lower both your hand and your leg. To ensure that your back is not drooping or stooped, check that it is still straight.

Reposition your eyes if you are experiencing discomfort in your neck.

- Continue doing the same with the other arm and leg. It is one repetition.

- **Seated lower back rotational stretch**

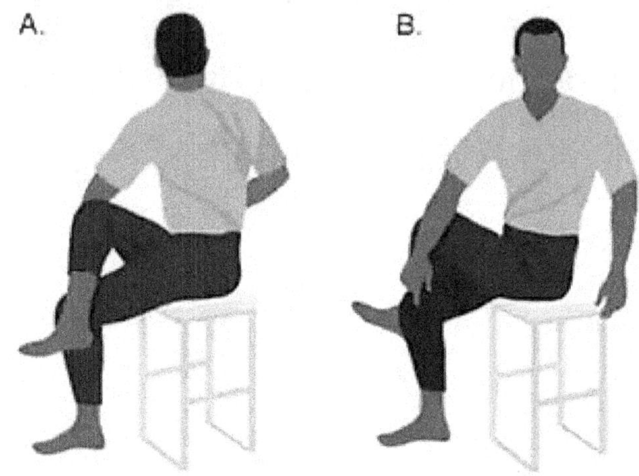

- Sit down on a stool or a chair that does not have arms.

- Lie down with your right leg crossed over your left leg.

- Twist and extend to the side while stabilizing your left elbow against the outside of your right knee during this exercise.

(A). Ten seconds should be held. On the other side, repeat the process.

(B). In a daily routine, perform this stretch three to five times on each side.

- **Shoulder blade squeeze**

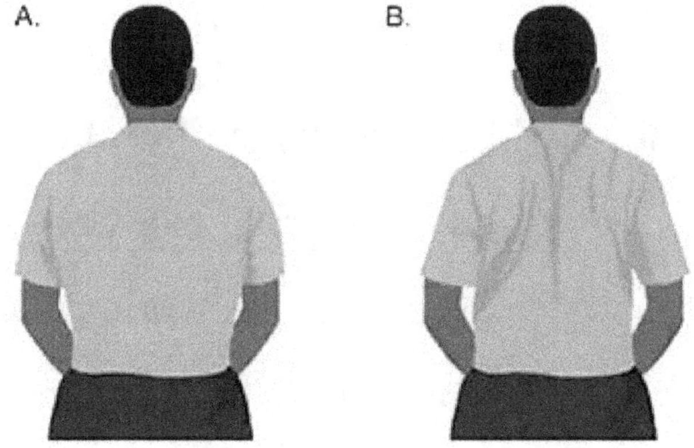

Sit on a stool or a chair that does not have arms (A). Holding your back straight, bring your shoulder blades together while you are seated (B). Keep this position for five seconds, and then let go. This should be done three to five times, twice a day.

# Conclusion

It is common for the symptoms of sciatica to improve on their own over time; however, certain sorts of activity may help the pain, while other types of movement may make the pain worse.

Stretching the hamstrings, performing specific abdominal strengthening exercises, and engaging in high-impact activities such as running and aerobics are all examples of the kind of workouts that have the potential to exacerbate the characteristics of sciatica.

It is possible to reduce the discomfort that is linked with sciatica by performing particular strengthening exercises, gentle stretching, and low-impact cardiovascular activities like To do

so, walking.